SAFE COUNSEL

A Complete Guide to Health Care and Home Remedies in the Late 19th Century

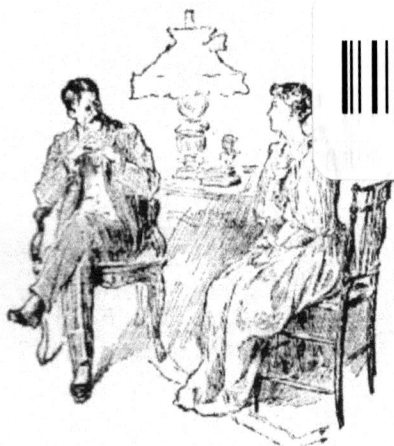

THE DOCTOR'S VISIT

ORIGINALLY PUBLISHED IN 1897

Edited by

Karen Hamilton Rager

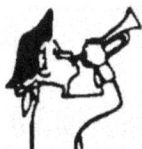

HERITAGE BOOKS
2011

HERITAGE BOOKS

AN IMPRINT OF HERITAGE BOOKS, INC.

Books, CDs, and more—Worldwide

For our listing of thousands of titles see our website
at
www.HeritageBooks.com

Published 2011 by
HERITAGE BOOKS, INC.
Publishing Division
100 Railroad Ave. #104
Westminster, Maryland 21157

Copyright © 2000 Karen Hamilton Rager

Other Heritage Books by the author:
*Safe Counsel: A Complete Guide to Pregnancy, Childbirth,
and Childcare in the Late 19th Century*

International Standard Book Numbers
Paperbound: 978-0-7884-1579-1
Clothbound: 978-0-7884-8933-4

TABLE OF CONTENTS

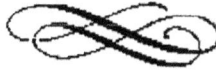

The Original Forward

1897

Knowledge is Safety

The old maxim, that "Knowledge is power," is a true one, but there is still a greater truth: "KNOWLEDGE IS SAFETY." Safety amid physical ills that beset mankind, and safety amid the moral pitfalls that surround so many young people, is the great crying demand of the age.

While the aim of this work, though novel and to some extent is daring, it is chaste, practical and to the point, and will be a boon and a blessing to thousands who consult its pages. The world is full of ignorance, and the ignorant will always criticize, because they love to suffer ills, for they know no better. New light is fast falling upon the dark corners, and the eyes of many are being opened.

The researches of science in the past few years have thrown light on many facts relating to the physiology of man and woman, and the diseases to which they are subject, and consequently many reformations have taken place in the treatment and prevention of diseases peculiar to the sexes.

Any information bearing upon the diseases of mankind should not be kept under lock and key. The physician is frequently called upon to speak in plain language to his patients upon some private and startling disease contracted on account of ignorance. The better plan, however, is to so educate and enlighten old and young upon the important subjects of health, so that the necessity to call a physician may occur less frequently.

A large, respectable, though diminishing class in every community, maintain that nothing that relates exclusively to either sex should become the subject of popular medical instruction. But such an opinion is radically wrong; ignorance is no more the mother of purity than it is of religion. Enlightenment can never work injustice to him who investigates.

The men and women who study and practice medicine are not the worse, but the better for such knowledge; so it would be to the community in general if all would be properly instructed on the laws of health which relate to the sexes.

Had every person a sound understanding on the relation of the sexes, one of the most fertile sources of crime and degradation would be removed. Physicians know too well what sad consequences are constantly occurring from a lack of proper knowledge on these important subjects.

Let the reader of this work study its pages carefully and be able to give safe counsel and advice to others, and remember that purity of purpose and purity of character are the brightest jewels in the crown of immortality.

Prof. B.G. Jefferis, M.D., PhD
1897

Chapter One

Celebrated Prescriptions for All Diseases and How to Use Them

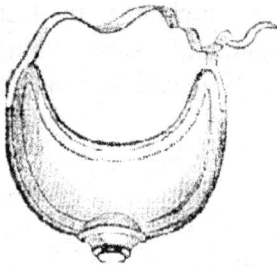

HOT-WATER THROAT BAG.   HOT-WATER BAG.

Amenorrhoea:

The following is recommended as a reliable emmenagogue in many cases of functional amenorrhoea:

    Bichloride of mercury
    Arsenite of sodium, aa gr. iij.
    Sulphate of strychnine, gr. iss
    Carbonate of potassium
    Sulphate of iron, aa gr. xlv.

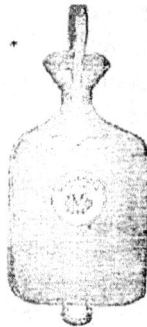

Mix and divide into sixty pills. Sig. One pill after each meal.

Apoplexy:

Occurs only in the corpulent or obese, and those of gross or high living.

Treatment: Raise the head to a barely upright position; loosen all tight clothes, strings, etc., and apply cold water to the head and warm water and warm cloths to the feet. Have the apartment cool and well ventilated. Give nothing by the mouth until the breathing is relieved, and then only draughts of cold water.

Bad Breath:

Bad or foul breath will be removed by taking a teaspoonful of the following mixture after each meal:

    one ounce chloride of soda
    one ounce liquor of potassa
    one and one-half ounces phosphate of soda
    three ounces of water

Biliousness:

Squeeze the juice of a lime or small lemon into half a glass of cold water, then stir in a little baking soda and drink while it foams. This recipe will also relieve sick headache if taken at the beginning.

Bilious Attacks:

Drop doses of muriatic acid in a wine glass of water every four hours, or the following prescription:

bicarbonate of soda, one drachm
aromatic spirits of ammonia, two drachms
peppermint water, four ounces

Dose: Take a teaspoonful every four hours.

Bites of Mad Dogs:

Apply caustic potash at once to the wound, and give enough whiskey to cause sleep.

Bleeding:

Very hot water is a prompt checker of bleeding, besides, if it is clean, as it should be, it aids in sterilizing the wound.

Boils:

These should be brought to a head by warm poultices of chamomile flowers, or boiled white lily root, or onion root, by fermentation with hot water, or by stimulating plasters. When ripe they should be destroyed by a needle or lancet. But this should not be attempted until they are thoroughly proved.

Bruises:

Apply the moist surface of the inside coating or skin of the shell of a raw egg. It will adhere of itself, leave no scar, and heal without pain.

Burns and Sores:

Pitch Burgundy, 2 pounds

Bees' Wax, 1 pound
Hog's lard, one pound

Mix all together and simmer over a slow fire until the whole are well mixed together; then stir it until cold. Apply on muslin to the parts affected.

Or:

Make a paste of common baking soda and water, and apply it promptly to the burn. It will quickly check the pain and inflammation.

Bunions:

May be checked in their early development by binding the joint with adhesive plaster, and keeping it on as long as any uneasiness is felt. The bandaging should be perfect, and it might be well to extend it round the foot. An inflamed bunion should be poulticed, and larger shoes be worn. Iodine 12 grains, lard or spermaceti ointment half an ounce, makes a capital ointment for bunions. It should be rubbed on gently twice or three times a day.

Chapped Hands:

Olive oil, 6 ounces
Camphor beat fine, 1/2 ounce

Mix, dissolve by gentle heat over slow fire and when cold apply to the hand freely.

When doing housework, if your hands become chapped or red, mix corn meal and vinegar into a stiff paste and apply to the hand two or three times a day, after washing them in hot water, then let dry without wiping, and rub with glycerine. At night use cold cream, and wear gloves.

Chicken Pox:

No medicine is usually needed, except a tea made from pleurisy root, to make the child sweat. Milk diet is the best; avoidance of animal food; careful attention to the bowels; keep cool and avoid exposure to cold.

Chilblains (also see Rheumatism):

One raw egg well beaten, half a pint of vinegar, one ounce spirits of turpentine, a quarter of an ounce of spirits of wine, a quarter of an ounce of camphor. These ingredients to be beaten together, then put in a bottle and shaken for ten minutes, after which, to be corked down tightly to exclude the air. In half an hour it is fit for use. To be well rubbed in, two, three, or four times a day. For rheumatism in the head, to be rubbed at the back of the neck and behind the ears. In chilblains this remedy is to be used before they are broken.

Colds on the Chest:

A flannel rag wrung out in boiling water and sprinkled with turpentine, laid on the chest, gives the greatest relief.

Colic:

Castor oil, given as soon as the symptoms of colic manifest themselves, has frequently afforded relief. At any rate, the irritating substances may be expelled from the alimentary canal before the pains will subside. All local remedies will be ineffectual, and consequently the purgative should be given in large doses until a copious vacuation is produced.

Cough:

Boil one ounce of flaxseed in a pint of water, strain, and add a little honey, one ounce of rock candy, and the juice of three lemons. Mix and boil well. Drink as hot as possible.

Coughs and Colds:

syrup of morphia, three ounces
syrup of tar, three and a half ounces
chloroform, one troy ounce
glycerine, one troy ounce.

Mix them. Dose, a teaspoonful three or four times a day.

Cramp:

Wherever friction can be conveniently applied, heat will be generated by it, and the muscle again reduced to a natural condition; but if the pains proceed from the contraction of some muscle located internally, burnt brandy is an excellent remedy.

A severe attack which will not yield to this simple treatment may be conquered by administering a small dose of laudanum or ether, best given under medical supervision.

Cuts (also see bruises):

A drop or two of creosote on a cut will stop its bleeding.

Deafness:

Obtain pure pickerel oil, and apply four drops morning and evening to the ear. Great care should be taken to obtain oil that is perfectly pure.

Also: Take three drops of sheep's gall, warm, and drop it into the ear on going to bed. The ear must be syringed with warm soap and water in the morning. The gall must be applied for three successive nights. It is only efficacious when the deafness is produced by cold. The most convenient way of warming the gall is by holding it in a silver spoon over the flame of a light. The above remedy has been frequently tried with perfect success.

Diarrhea:

The following prescription is generally all that will be necessary:

    acetate of lead, eight grains
    gum arabic, two drachms
    acetate of morphia, one grain
    cinnamon water, eight ounces

Take a teaspoonful every three hours. Be careful not to eat too much food. Some consider the best treatment is to fast, and it is a good suggestion. Patients should keep quiet and have the room of a warm and even temperature.

Disinfectant:

Chloride of lime should be scattered at least once a week under sinks and wherever sewer gas is likely to penetrate.

Dyspepsia:

> powdered rhubarb, two drachms
> bicarbonate of sodium, six drachms
> fluid extract of gentian, three drachms
> peppermint water, seven and a half ounces.

Mix them.   Dose, a teaspoonful half an hour before meals.

Eye Wash:

> Acetate of zinc, 20 grains
> Acetate of morphia, 5 grains
> Rose water, 4 ounces.

Mix.

Films and Cataracts of the Eyes:

> Blood Root Pulverized, 1 ounce
> Hog's lard, 3 ounces

Mix, simmer for 20 minutes, then strain; when cold put a little in the eyes twice or three times a day.

Foreign Body in the Eye:

When any foreign body enters the eye, close it instantly, and keep it still until you have an opportunity to ask the assistance of some one; then have the upper lid folded over a pencil and the exposed surfaces closely searched; if the body be invisible, catch the everted lid by the lashes, and drawing it down over the lower lid, suddenly release it, and it will resume its natural position. Unsuccessful in this attempt, you may be pretty well assured that the object has become lodged in the tissues, and will require assistance of a skilled operator to remove it.

Gout (also see rheumatism):

Commonly called in England the "Chelsea Pensioner"

half an ounce of nitre (saltpetre)
half an ounce of Sulphur
half an ounce of flour of mustard
half an ounce of turkey rhubarb
quarter of an ounce of powdered guaicum

Mix, and take a teaspoonful every other night for three nights, and omit three nights, in a wine-glassful of cold water which has been previously well boiled.

Headache:

Take a spoonful of finely powdered charcoal in a small glass of warm water to relieve a sick headache. It absorbs the gasses produced by the fermentation of undigested food.

Also: Gather sumach leaves in the summer, and spread them in the sun a few days to dry. Then powder them fine, and smoke, morning and evening for two weeks, also whenever there are symptoms of approaching headache. Use a new clay pipe. If these directions are adhered to, this medicine will surely effect a permanent cure.

Heartburn:

If soda, taken in small quantities after meals, does not relieve the distress, one may rest assured that the fluid is an alkali and requires an acid treatment. Proceed, after eating, to squeeze ten drops of lemon-juice into a small quantity of water, and swallow it. The habit of daily life should be made to conform to the laws of health, or local treatment will prove futile.

Hives:

After trying many remedies in a severe case of hives, Mr. Swain found vinegar lotion gave instant relief, and subsequent trials in other cases have been equally successful. One part of water to two parts of vinegar is the strength most suitable.

Also: Compound syrup of Squill, U.S., three ounces
Syrup of ipecac, U.S., one ounce

Mix them. Dose, a teaspoonful.

Insect Bites and Stings:

Wash with a solution of ammonia water.

Intoxication:

A man who is helplessly intoxicated may almost immediately restore the faculties and powers of locomotion by taking half a teaspoonful of chloride of ammonium in a goblet of water. A wineglassful of strong vinegar will have the same effect and is frequently resorted to by drunken soldiers.

Mashed Nails:

If the injured member be plunged into very hot water the nail will become pliable and adapt itself to the new condition of things, thus alleviating agony to some extent. A small hole may be bored on the nail with a pointed instrument, so adroitly so as not to cause pain, yet so successfully as to relieve pressure on the sensitive tissues. free applications of arnica or iodine will have an excellent effect.

Mumps:

It is very important that the face and neck be kept warm. Avoid catching cold, and regulate the stomach and bowels; because, when aggravated, this disease is communicated to other glands, and assumes there a serious form. Rest and quiet, with a good condition of the general health, will throw off this disease without further inconvenience.

Nervous Disability, Headache, Neuralgia, Nervousness:

Fluid extract of skullcap, 1 ounce
Fluid extract American valerian, 1 ounce
Fluid extract catnip, 1 ounce

Mix all. Dose, form 15 to 30 drops every two hours, in water; most valuable. A valuable tonic in all conditions of debility and want of appetite. Comp. tincture of cinchona in teaspoonful doses in little water, half hour before meals.

Neuralgia:

>   tincture of belladonna, one ounce
>   tincture of camphor, one ounce
>   tincture of arnica, one ounce
>   tincture of opium, one ounce

Mix them. Apply over the seat of the pain, and give ten to twenty drops in sweetened water every two hours.

Another Excellent Tonic:

>   Tincture of gentian, 1 ounce
>   Tincture of Columba, 1 ounce
>   Tincture of collinsonia, 1 ounce

Mix all. dose, one tablespoonful in one tablespoonful of water before meals.

Nose Bleeds:

May generally be stopped by putting a plug of lint into the nostril; if this does not do, apply a cold lotion to the forehead; raise the head and place both arms over the head, so that it will rest on both hands; dip the lint plug, slightly moistened, in some powdered gum arabic, and plug the nostrils again; or dip the plug into equal parts of gum arabic and alum. An easier and simpler method is to place a piece of writing paper on the gums of the upper jaw, under the upper lip, and let remain there for a few minutes.

Piles:

Hamamelis, both internally or as an injection in rectum. Bathe the parts with cold water or with astringent lotions, as alum water, especially in bleeding piles. Ointment of gallic acid and calomel is of repute. The best treatment of all is, suppositories of iodoform, ergotine, or tannic acid, which can be made at any drug store.

Poison Oak, Poison Ivy, Poison Sumach:

Frequent bathing of the affected parts in water as hot as can be borne are called for. If used immediately after exposure, it may prevent the eruption appearing. If later, it allays the itching, and gradually dries up the swellings, though they are very stubborn after they have once appeared. But an application every few hours keeps down the intolerable itching, which is the most annoying feature of sumach poisoning. In addition to this, the ordinary astringent ointments are useful, as is also that sovereign lotion, "lead water and laudanum".

Prickly Heat:

Caused by hot weather, by excess of flesh, by rough flannels, by sudden changes of temperature, or by over-fatigue.

Treatment: Bathe two or three times a day with warm water, in which a moderate quantity of bran and common soda has been stirred. After wiping the skin dry, dust the affected parts with common corn starch.

Quinsy:

An inflammation of the tonsils, or common inflammatory sore throat; commences with a slight feverish attack, with considerable pain and swelling of the tonsils, causing some difficulty in swallowing; as the attack advances, these symptoms become more intense, there is headache, thirst, a painful sense of tension, and acute darting pains in the ears. The attack is generally brought on by exposure to cold, and lasts from five to seven days, when it subsides naturally, or an abscess may form in tonsils and burst, or the tonsils may remain enlarged, the inflammation subsiding.

Treatment: The patient should remain in a warm room, the diet chiefly milk and good broths, some cooling laxative and diaphoretic medicine may be given; but the greatest relief will be found in the frequent inhalation of the steam of hot water through an inhaler, or in the old fashioned way through the spout of a teapot.

Rose Rash:

It requires no treatment except hygienic. Keep the bowels open. Nourishing diet, and if there is itching, moisten the skin with five per cent solution of aconite or solution of starch and water.

Ringworm:

The head is to be washed twice a day with soft soap and warm soft water; when dried the places to be rubbed with a piece of linen rag dipped in ammonia from gas tar; the patient should take a little Sulphur and molasses, or some other genuine aperient, every morning; brushes and combs should be washed every day, and the ammonia kept tightly corked.

Rheumatism (also see Gout):

One raw egg well beaten, half a pint of vinegar, one ounce spirits of turpentine, a quarter of an ounce of spirits of wine, a quarter of an ounce of camphor. These ingredients to be beaten together, then put in a bottle and shaken for ten minutes, after which, to be corked down tightly to exclude the air. In half an hour it is fit for use. To be well rubbed in, two, three, or four times a day.

Scarlet Fever:

Cold water compress on the throat. Fats and oils rubbed on hands and feet. The temperature of the room should be about 68 degrees Fahr., and all draughts avoided. Mustard baths for retrocession of the rash and to bring it out. Diet: ripe fruit, toast, gruel, beef tea and milk. Stimulants are useful to counteract depression of the vital forces.

Sore Throat (See Quinsy)

Sprains:

Wash the injury very frequently with cold salt and water, which is far better than warm vinegar or decoctions of herbs. Keep the injured limb as cool as possible to prevent inflammation, and sit with it elevated on a high cushion. Live on low diet, and take every morning some cooking medicine, such as Epsom salts. It cures in a few days.

Stabs:

A wound made by thrusting a dagger or other oblong instrument into the flesh, is best treated, if no artery has been severed, by applying lint scraped from a linen cloth, which serves as an obstruction, allowing and assisting coagulation.

Meanwhile cold water should be applied to the parts adjoining the wound.

Superfluous Hair:

> To remove superfluous hair
> sulphuret of arsenic, one ounce
> quicklime, one ounce
> prepared lard, one ounce
> white wax, one ounce

Melt the wax, add the lard. When nearly cold, stir in the other ingredients. Apply to the superfluous hair, allowing it to remain on from five to ten minutes; use a table-knife to shave off the hair; then wash with soap and warm water.

Sweating Feet, with Bad Odor:

Wash the feet in warm water with borax, and if this don't cure, use a solution of permanganate to destroy the fetor; about five grains to each ounce of water.

Throat Trouble:

A teaspoonful of salt, in a cup of hot water, makes a safe and excellent gargle in most throat troubles.

Turpentine Applications:

Mix turpentine and lard in equal parts. Warmed and rubbed on the chest, it is a safe, reliable and mild counter irretant and revulsant in minor lung complications.

Vomiting:

Ice dissolved in the mouth, often cures vomiting when all remedies fail. Much depends on the diet of persons liable to such attacks; this should be easily digestible food, taken often and in small quantities. Vomiting can often be arrested by applying a mustard paste over the region of the stomach. It is not necessary to allow it to remain until the parts are blistered, but it may be removed when the part becomes thoroughly red, and reapplied if required after the redness has disappeared. One of the secrets to relive vomiting is to give the stomach perfect rest, not allowing the patient even a glass of water, as long as the tendency remains to throw it up again.

Warts:

The easiest way to get rid of warts, is to pare off the thickened skin which covers the prominent wart; cut it off by successive layers and shave it until you come to the surface to the skin, and till you draw blood in two or three places. then rub the part thoroughly over with lunar caustic, and one effective operation of this kind will generally destroy the wart; if not, you cut off the black spot which has been occasioned by the caustic, and apply it again; or you may apply acetic acid, and thus you will get rid of it. Care must be taken in applying these acids, not to rub them on the skin around the wart.

Whooping Cough:

Dissolve a scruple of salt of tartar in a gill of water; add to it ten grains of cochineal; sweeten it with sugar. Give to an infant a quarter teaspoonful four times a day; two years old, on-half teaspoonful; from four years, a tablespoonful. Great care is required in the administration of medicines to infants. We can assure paternal inquirers that the foregoing may be depended upon.

Chapter Two

How to Cook for the Sick: Useful Dietetic Recipes

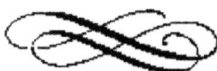

Apple Snow:

Take seven apples, not very sweet ones, and bake till soft and brown. Then remove the skins and cores; when cool, beat them smooth and fine; add one-half cup of granulated sugar and the white of one egg. Beat till the mixture will hold on your spoon. Serve with soft custard.

Apple Tapioca Pudding:

Soak a teacup of tapioca in a quart of warm water three hours. Cut in thin slices six tart apples, stir them lightly with the tapioca, add half cup sugar. Bake three hours. To be eaten with whipped cream. Good either warm or cold.

Apple Water:

Cut two large apples into slices and pour a quart of boiling water on them, or on roasted apples; strain in two or three hours and sweeten slightly.

Cream Gruel:

Put a pint and a half of water on the stove in a sauce pan. Take one tablespoon of flour and the same of cornmeal;

mix this with cold water, and as soon as the water in the sauce pan boils, stir it in slowly. Let it boil slowly about twenty minutes, stirring constantly; then add a little salt and a gill of sweet cream. Do not let it boil after putting in the cream, but turn into a bowl and cover tightly. Serve in a pretty cup and saucer.

Beef Tea:

For every quart of tea desired use one pound of fresh beef, from which all fat, bones and sinews have been carefully removed; cut the beef into pieces a quarter of an inch thick and mix with a pint of cold water. Let it stand an hour, then pour into a glass fruit can and place in a vessel of water; let it heat on the stove another hour, but do not let it boil. Strain before using.

Beef Tea and Oatmeal:

Beat two tablespoonfuls of fine oatmeal, with two tablespoonfuls of cold water until very smooth, then add a pint of hot beef tea. Boil together six or eight minutes, stirring constantly. Strain through a fine sieve.

Bread Jelly:

Pour boiling water over bread crumbs; place the mixture on the fire and let it boil until it is perfectly smooth. Take it off, and after pouring off the water, flavor with something

agreeable, as a little raspberry or currant jelly water. Pour into a mold until required for use.

Browned Rice:

Parch or brown rice slowly. Steep in milk for two hours. The rice or the milk only is excellent in summer complaint.

Chicken Jelly:

Take half a raw chicken, tie in a coarse cloth and pound, till well mashed, bones and meat together. Place the mass in a covered dish with water sufficient to cover it well. Allow it to simmer slowly till the liquor is reduced about one-half and the meat is thoroughly cooked. Press through a fine sieve or cloth, and salt to taste. Place on the stove to simmer about five minutes. When cold remove all particles of grease.

Cracked Wheat Pudding:

In a deep two-quart pudding dish put layers of cold, cooked, cracked wheat, and tart apples sliced thin, with four tablespoonfuls of sugar. Raisins can be added if preferred. fill the dish, having the wheat last, add a cup of cold water. Bake two hours.

Eggs (boiled):

An egg should never be boiled. Place in boiling water and set back on the stove for from seven to ten minutes. A little experience will enable anyone to do it successfully.

Egg Cocoa:

One-half teaspoon cocoa with enough hot water to make

21

a paste. Take one egg, beat white and yoke separately. Stir into a cup of milk heated to nearly boiling. Seeten if desired. Very nourishing.

Egg Lemonade:

White of one egg, one tablespoonful pulverized sugar, juice of one lemon and one goblet of water. Beat together. Very grateful in inflammation of lungs, stomach or bowels.

Eggs on Toast:

Soften brown bread toast with hot water, put on a platter and cover with poached or scrambled eggs.

Flaxseed Lemonade:

Two tablespoonfuls of whole flaxseed to a pint of boiling water, let it steep three hours, strain when cool and add the juice of two lemons and two tablespoonfuls of honey. If too thick, put in cold water. Splendid for colds and suppression of urine.

Fruit Blanc Mange:

One quart of juice of strawberries, cherries, grapes or other juicy fruit; one cup water. When boiling, add two tablespoonfuls sugar and four tablespoons cornstarch wet in cold water; let boil five or six minutes, then mold in small cups. Serve without sauce, or with cream or boiled custard. Lemon juice can be used the same, only requiring more water.

This is a very valuable dish for convalescents and pregnant women, where the stomach rejects solid food.

Graham Crisps:

Mix graham flour and cold water into a very stiff dough. Knead, roll very thin, and bake quickly in a hot oven. Excellent food for dyspeptics.

Graham Muffins:

Take one pint of new milk, one pint graham or entire wheat flour; stir together and add one beaten egg. Can be baked in any kind of gem pans or muffin rings. Salt must not be used with any bread that is made light with egg.

Hot Lemonade:

Take two thin slices and the juice of one lemon; mix with two tablespoonfuls of granulated sugar, and add one-half pint of boiling water.

Jelly Water:

Sour jellies dissolved in water make a pleasant drink for fever patients.

Lemon Jelly:

Moisten two tablespoonfuls of cornstarch, stir into one pint boiling water; add the juice of two lemons and one-half cup of sugar. Grate in a little of the rind. Put in molds to cool.

Milk Gruel:

Into a pint of scalding milk stir two tablespoonfuls of fine oatmeal. Add a pint of boiling water, and boil until the meal is thoroughly cooked.

Milk Porridge:

Place over the fire equal parts of milk and water. Just before it boils, add a small quantity (a tablespoonful to a pint of water) of graham flour or cornmeal, previously mixed with water, and boil three minutes.

Mulled Jelly:

Take one tablespoonful of currant or grape jelly; beat it with the white of one egg and a little loaf sugar; pour on it one-half pint of boiling water and break in a slice of dry toast or two crackers.

Oatmeal Gruel:

Stir two tablespoonfuls of coarse oatmeal into a quart of boiling water, and let it simmer two hours. Strain, if preferred.

Orangeade:

Take the thin peel of two oranges and of one lemon; add water and sugar the same as for hot lemonade. When cold add the juice of four or five oranges and one lemon and strain off.

Oysters (broiled):

Put large oysters on a wire toaster. Hold over hot coals until heated through. Serve on toast moistened with cream. Very grateful in convalescence.

Oysters (stewed):

Take one pint of milk, one cup of water, a teaspoon of salt; when boiling put in one pint of bulk oysters. Stir occasionally and remove from the stove before it boils. An oyster should not be shriveled in cooking.

Oyster Toast:

Pour stewed oysters over graham gems or bread toasted. Excellent for breakfast.

Pie for Dyspeptics:

Four tablespoonfuls of oatmeal, one pint of water; let stand for a few hours, or until the meal is swelled. then add two large apples, pared and sliced, a little salt, one cup of sugar, one tablespoonful of flour. Mix all well together and bake in a buttered dish; makes a most delicious pie, which can be eaten with safety by the sick or well.

Rice:

Take two cups of rice and one and one-half pints of milk. Place in a covered dish and steam in a kettle of boiling water until it is cooked through, pour into cups and let it stand until cold. Serve with cream.

Rice Omelet:

Two cups boiled rice, one cup sweet milk, two eggs. Stir together with egg beater, and put into a hot buttered skillet. Cook slowly ten minutes, stirring frequently.

Sago Gruel:

Take two tablespoons of sago and place them in a small saucepan, moisten gradually with a little cold water. Set the preparation on a slow fire, and keep stirring till it becomes rather stiff and clear. Add a little grated nutmeg and sugar to taste; if preferred, half a pat of butter may also be added with the sugar.

Sago Jelly:

Simmer gently in a pint of water two tablespoonfuls of sago until it thickens, frequently stirring. A little sugar may be added if desired.

Strawberry Dessert:

Place alternate layers of hot cooked cracked wheat and strawberries in a deep dish; when cold, turn out on platter; cut in slices and serve with cream and sugar, or strawberry juice. Wet the molds with cold water before using. This, molded in small cups, makes a dainty dish for the sick. Wheatlet can be used in the same way.

Toast Water:

Toast several thin pieces of bread a nice deep brown, but do not blacken or burn. Break into small pieces and put into a jar. Pour over the pieces a quart of boiling water; cover the jar and let it stand an hour before using. Strain if desired.

White of Egg and Milk:

The white of an egg beaten to a stiff froth, and stirred very quickly into a glass of milk, is a very nourishing food for persons whose digestion is weak, also for children who cannot digest milk alone.

Sensible Rules for the Nurse

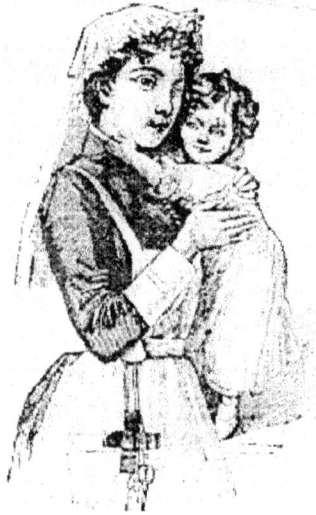

Remember to be extremely neat in dress; a few drops of hartshorn in the water used for *daily* bathing will remove the disagreeable odors of warmth and perspiration.

Never speak of the symptoms of your patient in his presence, unless questioned by the doctor, whose orders you are always to obey *implicitly*.

Remember never to be a gossip or tattler, and always to hold sacred the knowledge which, to a certain extent, you must obtain of the private affairs of your patient and the household in which you nurse.

Never contradict your patient, nor argue with him, nor let him see that you are annoyed about anything.

Never *whisper* in the sick room. If your patient be well enough, and wishes you to talk to him, speak in a low, distinct voice, on cheerful subjects. Don't relate painful hospital experiences, nor give details of the maladies of former patients, and remember never to startle him with accounts of dreadful crimes or accidents that you have read in the newspapers.

Write down the orders that the physician gives you as to time for giving the medicines, food, etc.

Keep the room bright (unless the doctor orders it darkened).

Let the air of the room be as pure as possible, and keep everything in order, but without being fussy and bustling.

The only way to remove dust in a sick room is to wipe everything with a damp cloth.

Remember to carry out all vessels covered. Empty and wash them immediately, and keep some disinfectant in them.

Remember that to leave the patient's untasted food by his side, from meal to meal, in hopes that he will eat it in the interval, is simply to prevent him from taking any food at all.

Medicines, beef tea or stimulants, should never be kept where the patient can see them or smell them.

Light-colored clothing should be worn by those who have the care of the sick, in preference to dark-colored apparel; particularly if the disease is of a contagious nature. Experiments have shown that black and other dark colors will absorb more readily the subtle effluvia that emanates from sick persons than white or light colors.

Safe Counsel

Longevity

The following table exhibits very recent mortality statistics, showing the average duration of life among persons of various classes:

Employment.	*Years.*
Judges	65
Farmers	64
Bank Officers	64
Coopers	58
Public Officers	57
Clergymen	56
Shipwrights	55
Hatters	54
Lawyers	54
Rope Makers	54
Blacksmiths	51
Merchants	51
Calico Printers	51
Physicians	51
Butchers	50
Carpenters	49
Masons	48
Traders	46
Tailors	44
Jewelers	44
Manufacturers	43
Bakers	43
Painters	43
Shoemakers	43
Mechanics	43
Editors	40
Musicians	39
Printers	38
Machinists	36
Teachers	34
Clerks	34
Operatives	32

"It will be easily seen, by these figures, how a quiet or tranquil life affects longevity. The phlegmatic man will live longer, all other things being equal, than the sanguine, nervous individual. Marriage is favorable to longevity, and it has also been ascertained that women live longer than men."

Chapter Three
Practical Rules for Bathing

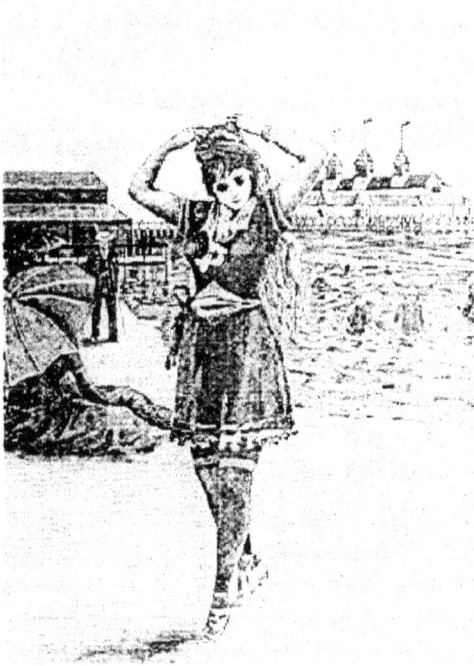

Bathe at least once a week all over, thoroughly. No one can preserve his health by neglecting personal cleanliness. Remember, "Cleanliness is akin to Godliness."

Only mild soap should be used in bathing the body.

Wipe quickly and dry the body thoroughly with a moderately coarse towel. Rub the skin vigorously.

Many people have contracted severe and fatal diseases by neglecting to take proper care of the body after bathing.

If you get up a good reaction by thorough rubbing in a mild temperature, the effect is always good.

Never go into a cold room, or allow cold air to enter the room until you are dressed.

Bathing in cold rooms and in cold water, is positively injurious, unless the person possesses a very strong and vigorous constitution, and then there is great danger of laying the foundation of some serious disease.

Never bathe within two hours after eating. It injures digestion.

Never bathe when the body or mind is much exhausted. It is liable to check the healthful circulation.

A good time for bathing is just before retiring. The morning hour is a good time also, if a warm room and warm water can be secured.

Never bathe a fresh wound or broken skin with cold water; the wound absorbs water, and causes swelling and irritation.

A person not robust should be very careful in bathing; great care should be exercised to avoid any chilling effects.

The Different Kinds of Baths, and How to Prepare Them

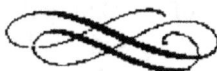

Acid Bath:

Place a little vinegar in water, and heat to the usual temperature. This is an excellent remedy for the disorders of the liver.

Foot Bath:

The foot-bath, in coughs, colds, asthma, headaches and fevers, is excellent. One or two table-spoonfuls of ground mustard added to a gallon of hot water, is very beneficial. Heat the water as hot as the patient can endure it, and gradually increase the temperature by pouring in additional quantities of hot water during the bath.

Hot-Air Bath:

Place the alcohol lamp under the chair, without the dish of water. Then place the patient on the chair, as in the vapor bath, and let him remain until a gentle and free perspiration is produced. This bath may be taken from time to time as may be deemed necessary.

While remaining in the hot-air bath the patient may drink freely of cold or tepid water. As soon as the bath is over the patient should be washed with hot water and soap. The hot-air bath is excellent for colds, skin diseases, and the gout.

Salt Bath:

To open the pores of the skin, put a little common salt into the water. Borax, baking soda or lime used in the same way are excellent for cooling and cleansing the skin. A very small quantity in a bowl is sufficient.

Sitz Bath:

A tub is arranged so that the patient can sit down in it while bathing. Fill the tub about one-half full of water. This is an excellent remedy for piles, constipation, headache, gravel, and for acute and inflammatory affections generally.

Sponge Bath:

Have a large basin of water of the temperature of 88 or 95 degrees. As soon as the patient rises rub the body over with a soft, dry towel until it becomes warm. Now sponge the body with water and a little soap, at the same time keeping the body well covered, except such portions as are necessarily exposed. Then dry the skin well for two or three minutes, until every part becomes red and perfectly dry.

Sulphur, lime or salt, and sometimes mustard, may be used in any of the sponge-baths, according to the disease.

Sulphur Bath:

For the itch, ringworm, itching, and for other slight skin irritations, bathe in water containing a little Sulphur.

Vapor Bath:

For catarrh, bronchitis, pleurisy, inflammation of the lungs, rheumatism, fever, affections of the bowels and kidneys, and skin diseases, the vapor-bath is an excellent remedy.

Use a small alcohol lamp, and place over it a small dish containing water. Light the lamp and allow the water to boil. Place a cane-bottom chair over the lamp and seat the patient on it. Wrap blankets or quilts around the chair and around the patient, closing it tightly about the neck. After free perspiration is produced the patient should be wrapped in warm blankets, and placed in bed, so as to continue the perspiration for some time.

A convenient alcohol lamp may be made by taking a tin box, placing a tube in it, and putting in a common lamp wick. Any tinner can make one in a few minutes, at a trifling cost.

Chapter Four

The Toilet

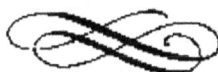

Important Rules. - The first care of all persons should be for their personal appearance. Those who are slovenly or careless in their habits are unfit for refined society, and cannot possibly make a good appearance in it. A well-bred person will always cultivate habits of the most scrupulous neatness. A gentleman or lady is always well-dressed. The garment may be plain or of coarse material or even worn "thin and shiny," but if it is carefully brushed and neat, it can be worn with dignity.

Personal Cleanliness. - The first point which marks the gentleman or lady in appearance is rigid cleanliness. This remark supplies to the body and everything which covers it. A clean skin - only to be secured by frequent baths - is indispensable.

The Teeth. - The teeth should receive the utmost attention. Many a young man has been disgusted with a lady by seeing her unclean and discolored teeth. It takes but a few moments, and if necessary secure some simple tooth powder or rub the teeth thoroughly every day with a linen handkerchief, and it will give the teeth and mouth a beautiful and clean appearance.

The Hair and Beard. - The hair should be thoroughly brushed and well kept, and the beard of men properly trimmed. Men should not let their hair grow long and shaggy.

Underclothing. - The matter of cleanliness extends to all articles of clothing, underwear as well as the outer-clothing. Some persons have an odor about them that is very offensive, simply on account of their underclothing being worn too long without washing.

The Bath. - A bath should be taken at least once a week, and if the feet perspire they should be washed several times a week, as the case may require. It is not unfrequent that young men are seen with dirty ears and neck. This is unpardonable and boorish, and shows gross neglect.

Soiled Garments. - A young man's garments may not be expensive, yet there is no excuse for wearing a soiled collar and a soiled shirt, or carrying a soiled handkerchief. No one should appear as though he had slept in a stable, shaggy hair, soiled clothing or garments indifferently put on and carelessly buttoned. A young man's vest should always be kept buttoned in the presence of ladies.

The Breath. - Care should be taken to remedy an offensive breath without delay. Nothing renders one so unpleasant to one's acquaintance, or is such a source of misery to one's self. The evil may be from some derangement of the stomach or some defective condition of the teeth, or catarrhal affection of the throat and nose.

Sensible helps to Beauty

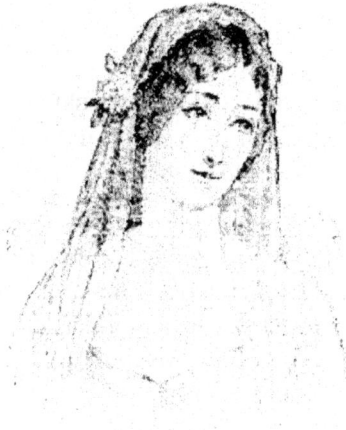

For **Scrawny Neck**. - Take off your tight collars, feather boas and such heating things. Wash neck and chest with hot water, then rub in sweet oil all that you can work in. Apply this every night before you retire and leave the skin damp with it while you sleep.

For **Red Hands**. - Keep your feet warm by soaking them often in hot water, and keep your hands out of the water as much as possible. Rub your hands with the skin of a lemon and it will white them. If your skin will bear glycerine after you have washed, pour into the palm a little glycerine and lemon juice mixed, and rub over the hands and wipe off.

Neck and Face. - Do not bathe the neck and face just before or after being out of doors. It tends to wrinkle the skin.

Scowls. - Never allow yourself to scowl, even if the sun be in your eyes. That scowl will soon leave its trace and no beauty will outlive it.

Wrinkled Forehead. - If you wrinkle your forehead when you talk or read, visit an oculist and have your eyes tested, and then wear glasses to fit them.

Old Looks. - Sometimes your face looks old because it is tired. Then apply the following wash and it will make you look younger: Put three drops of ammonia, a little borax, a tablespoon of bay rum, and a few drops of camphor into warm water and apply to your face. Avoid getting it into your eyes.

The Best Cosmetic. - Squeeze the juice of a lemon into a pint of sweet milk. Wash the face with it every night and in the morning wash off with warm rain water. This will produce a very beautiful effect upon the skin.

Spots on the Face. - Moles and many other discoloration's may be removed from the face by a preparation composed of one part chemically pure carbolic acid and two parts pure glycerine. Touch the spots with a camel's-hair pencil, being careful that the preparation does not come in contact with the adjacent skin. Five minutes after touching, bathe with soft water and apply a little vaseline. It may be necessary to repeat the operation, but if persisted in, the blemishes will be entirely removed.

Wrinkles. - This prescription is said to cure wrinkles: Take one ounce of white wax and melt it to a gentle heat. Add two ounces of the juice of lily bulbs, two ounces of honey, two drams of rose water, and a drop or two of ottar of roses. Apply twice a day, rubbing the wrinkles the wrong way. Always use tepid water for washing the face.

The Hair. - The hair must be kept free from dust or it will fall out. One of the best things for cleaning it, is a raw egg rubbed into the roots and then washed out in several waters. The egg furnishes material for the hair to grow on, while keeping the scalp perfectly clean. Apply once a month.

Loss of Hair. - When through sickness or headache the hair falls out, the following tonic may be applied with good effect: Use one ounce of glycerine, one ounce of bay rum, one pint of strong sage tea, and apply every other night, rubbing well into the scalp.

How to keep the bloom and grace of youth

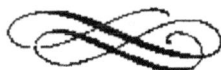

The Secret of its Preservation. - The question most often asked by women is regarding the art of retaining, with advancing years, the bloom and grace of youth. This secret is not learned through the analysis of chemical compounds, but by a thorough study of nature's laws peculiar to their sex.. There are truths, simple yet wonderful, whereby the bloom of early life can be restored and retained, as should be the heritage of all God's children, sending the light of beauty into every woman's face.

Hard Water. - Do not bathe in hard water; soften it with a few drops of ammonia, or a little borax.

Bathing the Face. - Do not bathe the face while it is very warm, and never use very cold water. Do not attempt to remove dust with cold water; give your face a hot bath, using plenty of good soap, then give it a thorough rinsing with warm water. Do not rub your face with a coarse towel.

Wrinkles. - Do not believe you can remove wrinkles by filling the crevices with powder. Give your face a Russian bath every night; that is, bathe it with water so hot that you wonder how you can bear it, and then, a minute after, with moderately cold water, that will make your face glow with warmth; dry it with a soft towel.

Chapter Five

Corsets

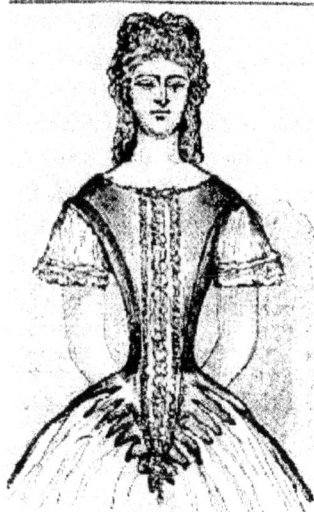

How to Determine a Perfect Human Figure

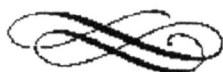

The proportions of the perfect human figures are strictly mathematical. The whole figure is six times the length of the foot. Whether the form be slender or plump, this rule holds good. The Greeks made all their statures according to this rule. The face, from the highest point of the forehead, where the hair begins, to the end of the chin, is one-tenth of the whole stature. The hand, from the wrist to the end of the middle finger, is the same. The chest is a fourth, and from the nipples to the top of the head is the same. From the top of the chest to the highest point of the forehead is a seventh. If the length of the face, from the roots of the hair to the chin, be divided into three equal parts, the first division determines the point where the eyebrows meet, and the second the place of the nostrils. The navel is the central point of the human body; and if a man should lie on his back with his arms and legs extended, the periphery of the circle which might be described around him, with the navel for its center, would touch the extremities of his hands and feet. The height from the feet to the top of the head is the same as the distance from the extremity of one hand to the extremity of the other when the arms are extended.

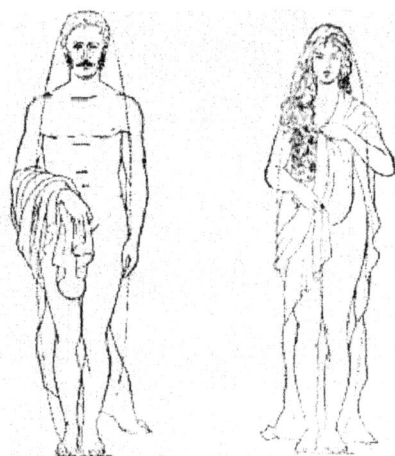

MALE.   FEMALE.
Showing the Difference in Form and Proportion.

The History, Mystery, Benefits and Injuries of the Corset

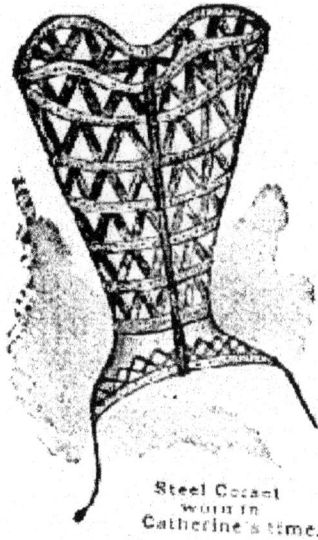

Steel Corset
worn in
Catherine's time.

The origin of the corset is lost in remote antiquity. The figures of the early Egyptian women show clearly an artificial shape of the waist produced by some style of corset. A similar style of dress must also have prevailed among the ancient Jewish maidens; for Isaiah, in calling upon the women to put away their personal adornments, says: "Instead of a girdle there shall be a rent, and instead of a stomacher (corset) a girdle of sackcloth."

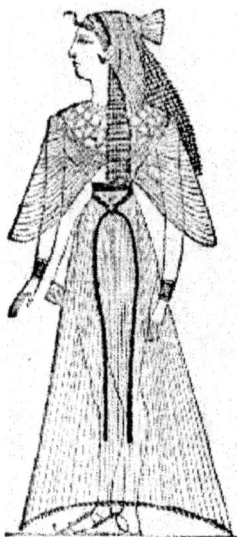

EGYPTIAN CORSET.

Homer also tells us of the cestus or girdle of Venus, which was borrowed by the haughty Juno with a view to increasing her personal attractions, that Jupiter might be a more tractable and orderly husband.

Coming down to the later times, we find the corset was used in France and England as early as the 12th century.

The most extensive and extreme use of the corset occurred in the 16th century, during the reign of Catherine de Medici of France and Queen Elizabeth of England. With Catherine de Medici a thirteen-inch waist measurement was considered the standard of fashion, while a thick waist was an abomination. No lady could consider her figure of proper shape unless she could span her waist with her two hands. To produce this result a strong rigid corset was worn night and day until the waist was laced down to the required size. Then over this corset was placed the steel apparatus shown in the illustration.

This corset-cover reached from the hip to the throat, and produced a rigid figure over which the dress would fit with perfect smoothness.

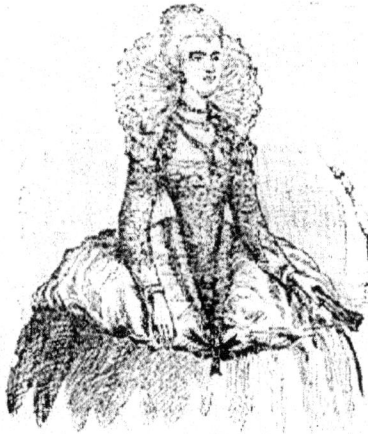

Forms of Corsets in the time of Elizabeth of England.

During the 18th century corsets were largely made from a species of leather known as "Bend", which was not unlike that used for shoe soles, and measured nearly a quarter of an inch in thickness.

About the time of the French Revolution a reaction set in against tight lacing and for a time there was a return to the early classical Greek costume.

This style of dress prevailed, with various modifications, until about 1810, when corsets and tight lacing again returned with threefold fury.

Buchan, a prominent writer of this period, says that it was by no means uncommon to see "a mother lay her daughter down upon the carpet, and, placing her foot upon her back, break half a dozen laces in tightening her stays."

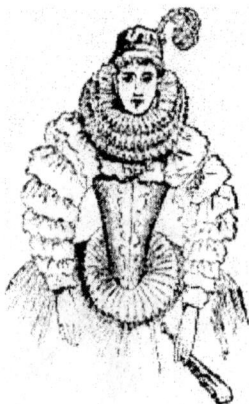

It is reserved to our own time to demonstrate that corsets and tight lacing do not necessarily go hand in hand. Distortion and feebleness are not beauty. A proper proportion should exist between the size of the waist and the breadth of the shoulders and hips, and if the waist is diminished below this proportion, it suggests disproportion and invalidism rather than grace and beauty.

The perfect corset is one which possesses just that degree of rigidity which will prevent it from wrinkling, but will at the same time allow freedom in the bending and twisting of the body. Corsets boned with whalebone, horn or steel are necessarily stiff, rigid and uncomfortable. After a few days' wear the bones or steels become bent and set in position, or, as more frequently happens, they break and cause injury or discomfort to the wearer.

About seven years ago (1888) an article was discovered for the stiffening of corsets, which has revolutionized the corset industry of the world. This article is manufactured from the natural fibers of the Mexican Ixtle plant, and is know as Coraline. It consists of straight, stiff fibers like bristles, bound together into a cord by being wound with two strands of thread passing in opposite directions.

This produces an elastic fiber intermediate in stiffness between twine and whalebone. It cannot break, but it possesses all the stiffness and flexibility necessary to hold the corset in shape and prevent its wrinkling.

We congratulate the ladies of to-day upon the advantages they enjoy over their sisters of two centuries ago, in the forms and the graceful and easy curves of the corsets now made as compared with those of former times.

The Effects of Tight-Lacing

It destroys natural beauty and creates an unpleasant and irritable temper. A tight-laced chest and a good disposition cannot go together.

The human form has been molded by nature, the best shape is undoubtedly that which she has given it. To endeavor to render it more elegant by artificial means is to change it; to make it much smaller below and much larger above is to destroy its beauty; to keep it cased up in a kind of domestic cuirass is not only to deform it, but to expose the internal parts to serious injury.

Under such compression as is commonly practiced by ladies, the development of the bones, which are still tender, does not take place conformably to the intention of nature, because nutrition is necessarily stopped, and they consequently become twisted and deformed.

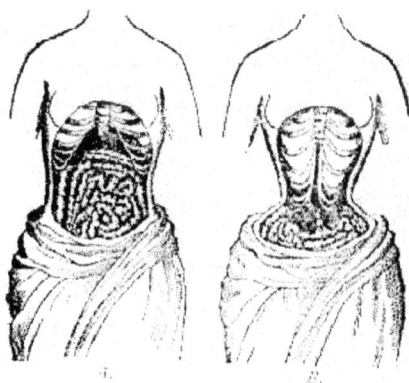

The ribs charge cures; the large lower rib very low down, across, all with absolute room.

The ribs bent almost to angles; the organs cramped, the liver, stomach and intestines forced down into the ilia, others in the womb seriously.

Nature Versus Corsets Illustrated

These who wear these appliances of tight-lacing often complain that they cannot sit upright without them - are sometimes, indeed, compelled to wear them during all the twenty-four hours; a fact which proves to what extent such articles weaken the muscles of the trunk.

The injury does not fall merely on the internal structure of the body, but also on its beauty, and on the temper and feelings with which that beauty is associated.

Chapter Six

The Care of the Hair

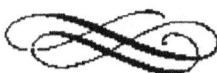

The Color of the Hair. - The color of the hair corresponds with that of the skin - being dark or black, with a dark complexion, and red or yellow with a fair skin. When a white skin is seen in conjunction with black hair, as among the women of Syria and Barbary, the apparent exception arises form protection from the sun's rays, and opposite colors are often found among people of one prevailing feature. Thus red-haired Jews are not uncommon, though the nation in general have dark complexion and hair.

The Imperishable Nature of Hair. - The imperishable nature of hair arises from the combination of salt and metals in it composition. In old tombs and on mummies it has been found in a perfect state, after a lapse of over two thousand years. There are many curious accounts proving the indestructibility of the human hair.

Tubular. - In the human family the hairs are tubular, the tubes being intersected by partitions, resembling in some degree the cellular tissue of plants. Their hollowness prevents imcumbrance form weight, while their powers of resistance is increased by having their traverse sections rounded in form.

Cautions. - It is ascertained that a full head of hair, beard and whiskers, are a prevention against colds and consumption's.

Occasionally, however, it is found necessary to remove the hair from the head, in cases of fever or disease, to stay the inflammatory symptoms, and to relieve the brain. The head should invariably be kept cool. Close night-caps are unhealthy, and smoking-caps and coverings for the head within doors are alike detrimental to the free growth of the hair, weakening it, and causing it to fall out.

How To Beautify and Preserve the Hair

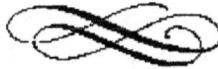

To Beautify the Hair

Keep the head clean, the pores of the skin open, and the whole circulatory system in a healthy condition, and you will have no need of bear's grease (alias hog's lard. Where there is a tendency in the hair to fall off on account of the weakness or sluggishness of the circulation, or an unhealthy state of the skin, cold water and friction with a tolerably stiff brush are probably the best remedial agents.

Barber's Shampoos

Carefully avoid all kinds of barber's shampoos, hair oils, etc. They are injurious and in time will ruin a good head of hair. Avoid strong shampoos of any kind.

Care of the Hair

To keep the hair healthy, keep the head clean. Brush the scalp well with a stiff brush, while dry. Then wash with castile soap, and rub into the roots, bay rum, brandy or camphor water. This done twice a month will prove beneficial. Brush the scalp thoroughly twice a week. Dampen the hair with soft water at the toilet, and do not use oil.

Hair Wash

Take one ounce of borax, half an ounce of camphor powder - these ingredients fine - and dissolve them in one quart of boiling water. When cool, the solution will be ready for use. Dampen the hair frequently. This wash is said not only to cleanse and beautify, but to strengthen the hair, preserve the color and prevent baldness.

Another Excellent Wash

The best wash we know for cleansing and softening the hair is an egg beaten up and rubbed well into the hair, and afterwards washed out with several washes of warm water.

The Only Sensible and Safe Hair Oil

The following is considered a most valuable preparation:

Extract of yellow Peruvian bark, fifteen grains
Extract of rhatany root, eight grains
Extract of burdoch root and oil of nutmegs (fixed) of each two drachms
Camphor (dissolve with spirits of wine), fifteen grains
Beef marrow, two ounces
Best olive oil, one ounce
Citron juice, half a drach
Aromatic essential oil, as mush as sufficient to render it fragrant: (Two drachms of bergamot, and a few drops of ottar of roses would suffice.)

Mix and make into an ointment.

Hair Wash

A good hair wash is soap and water, and the oftener it is applied the freer the surface of the head will be from scurf. The hair-brush should also be kept in requisition morning and evening.

To Remove Superfluous Hair

With those who dislike the use of arsenic, the following is used for removing superfluous hair from the skin:

> Lime, one ounce
> Carbonate of potash, two ounces
> Charcoal powder, one drachm

For use, make it into a paste with a little warm water, and apply it to the part, previously shaved close. As soon as it has become thoroughly dry, it may be washed off with a little warm water.

Coloring for Eyelashes and Eyebrows

In eyelashes the chief element of beauty consists in their being long and glossy; the eyebrows should be finely arched and clearly divided from each other. The most innocent darkener of the brow is the expressed juice of the elderberry, or a burnt clove.

Crimping Hair

To make the hair stay in crimps, take five cents worth of gum arabic and add to it just enough boiling water to dissolve it. When dissolved, add enough alcohol to make it rather thin. Let this stand all night and then bottle it to prevent the alcohol from evaporating. This put on the hair at night, after it is done up in papers or pins, will make it stay in crimp the hottest day, and is perfectly harmless.

To Curl the Hair

There is no preparation that will make naturally straight hair assume a permanent curl. The following will keep the hair in curl for a short time: Take borax, two ounces; gum arabic, one drachm; and hot water, not boiling, one quart; stir, and, as soon as the ingredients are dissolved, add three tablespoonfuls of strong spirits of camphor. On retiring to rest, wet the hair with the above liquid, and roll in twists of paper as usual. Do not disturb the hair until morning, then untwist and form into ringlets.

For Falling or Loosening of Hair

Take:

> Alcohol, a half pint
> Salt, as much as will dissolve
> Glycerine, a tablespoonful
> Flour of Sulphur, teaspoonful

Mix. Rub on the scalp every morning.

To Darken the Hair without Bad Effects

Take: Blue vitriol (powdered), one drachm

> Alcohol, one ounce
> Essence of roses, ten drops

Rain-water, a half pint

Shake together until they are thoroughly dissolved.

Gray Hair

There are no know means by which the hair can be prevented from turning gray, and none which can restore it to its original hue, except through the process of dyeing. The numerous "hair color restorers" which are advertised are chemical preparations which act in the manner of a dye or as a paint, and are nearly always dependent for their power on the presence of lead. This mineral, applied to the skin, for a long time, will lead to the most disastrous maladies - lead-palsy, lead colic, and other symptoms of poisoning. It should, therefore, never be used for this purpose.

Chapter Seven

Puberty & Sex

Puberty, Virility and Hygienic Laws

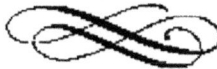

Proper Age

The proper age for puberty should vary from twelve to eighteen years. As a general rule, in the more vigorous and the more addicted to athletic exercise or out-door life, this change is slower in making its approach.

Hygienic Attention

Youths at this period should receive special private attention. They should be taught the purpose of the sexual organs and the proper hygienic laws that govern them, and they should also be taught to rise in the morning and not to lie in bed after waking up, because it is largely owing to this habit that the secret vice is contracted.

Masturbation

One of the common causes of premature excitement in many boys is a tight foreskin. It may cause much evil and ought always to be remedied. Ill-fitting garments often cause much irritation in children and produce unnatural passions. It is best to have boys sleep in separate beds and not have them sleep together if it can be avoided.

How to Cure Pimples or other Facial Eruptions

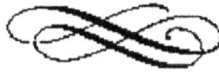

It requires self-denial to get rid of pimples, for persons troubled with them will persist in eating fat meats and other articles of food calculated to produce them. Avoid the use of rich gravies, or pastry, or anything of the kind in excess. Take all the our-door exercise you can and never indulge in a late supper. Retire at a reasonable hour, and rise early in the morning. Sulphur to purify the blood may be taken three times a week - a thimbleful in a glass of milk before breakfast. It takes some time for the Sulphur to do its work, therefore persevere in its use till the humors, or pimples, or blotches, disappear. Avoid getting wet while taking the Sulphur.

Try this Recipe

Wash the face twice a day in warm water, and rub dry with a coarse towel. Then with a soft towel rub in a lotion made of:

Two ounces of white brandy
One ounce of cologne
One-half ounce of liquor potassa

Persons subject to skin eruptions should avoid very salty or fat food. A dose of Epsom salts occasionally might prove beneficial.

Wash the face in a dilution of carbolic acid, allowing one teaspoonful to a pint of water. This is an excellent and purifying lotion, and may be used on the most delicate skins. Be careful about letting this wash get into the eyes.

Another recipe:

Oil of sweet almonds, one ounce
Fluid potash, one drachm

Shake well together, and then add:

rose water, one ounce
pure water, six ounces

Mix. Rub the pimples or blotches for some minutes with a rough towel, and then dab them with the lotion.

Or try this:

Dissolve one ounce of borax, and sponge the face with it every night. When there are insects, rub on flower of sulphar, dry after washing, rub well and wipe dry; use plenty of castile soap.

Another remedy:

Dilute corrosive sublimate with oil of almonds. a few days' application will remove them.

Masturbation

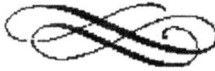

In some cases, the only complaint the patient will make on consulting you, is that he is suffering under a kind of continued fever. He will probably present a hot, dry skin, with something of a hectic appearance.

The sleep seems to be irregular and unrefreshing - restlessness during the early part of the night, and in the advanced stages of the disease, profuse sweats before morning. There is also frequent starting in the sleep, from disturbing dreams. The characteristic feature is, that your patient almost always dreams of sexual intercourse.

Other common symptoms are nervous headache, giddiness, ringing in the ears, and a dull pain in the back part of the head. It is frequently the case that the patient suffers a stiffness in the neck , darting pains in the forehead, and also weak eyes are among the common symptoms.

One very frequent, and perhaps early symptom (especially in young females) is solitariness - a disposition to seclude themselves from society. Although they may be tolerable cheerful when in company, they prefer rather to be alone.

The countenance has often a gloomy and worn-down expression. The patients friends frequently notice a great change. Large livid spots under the eyes is a common feature. Sudden flashes of heat may be noticed passing over the patient's face. He is liable also to palpitations. The pulse is

71

very variable generally too slow. Extreme emaciation, without any other assignable cause for it, may be set down as another very common symptom.

If the evil has gone on for several years, there will be a general unhealthy appearance, of a character so marked, as to enable an experienced observer at once to detect the cause. In the case of onanists especially there is a peculiar rank odor emitted from the body, by which they may be readily distinguished. One striking peculiarity of all these patients is that they cannot look a man in the face!

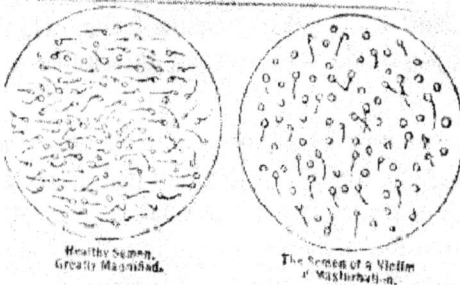

Healthy Semen.
Greatly Magnified.

The Semen of a Victim
of Masturbation.

Home Treatment of the Secret Habit

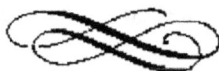

1. The first condition of recovery is a prompt and permanent abandonment of the ruinous habit.

2. Keep the mind employed by interesting the patient in the various topics of the day, and social features of the community.

3. Plenty of bodily out of door exercise, hoeing in the garden, walking, or working on the farm; of course not too heavy work must be indulged in.

4. If the patient is weak and very much emaciated, cod liver oil is an excellent remedy.

5. The patient should live principally on brown bread, oat meal, graham crackers, wheat meat, cracked or boiled wheat, or hominy, and food of that character. No meats should be indulged in whatever; milk diet if used by the patient is an excellent remedy. Plenty of fruit should be indulged in; dried toast and baked apples make an excellent supper. The patient should eat early in the evening, never late at night.

6. Avoid all tea, coffee, or alcoholic stimulants of any kind.

7. "Early to bed and early to rise," should be the motto of every victim of this vice. A patient should take a cold bath every morning after rising. A cold water injection in moderate quantities before retiring has cured many patients.

8. If the above remedies are not sufficient, a family physician should be consulted.

9. Never let children sleep together, if possible, to avoid it. Discourage the children of neighbors and friends from sleeping with your children.

10. Have your children rise early. It is the lying in bed in the morning that plays the mischief.

Nocturnal Emissions

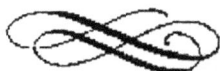

Involuntary emissions of semen during amorous dreams at night is not at all uncommon among healthy men. When this occurs from one to three or four times a month, no anxiety or concern need be felt.

When the emissions take place without dreams, manifested only by stained spots in the morning on the linen, or take place at stool and are entirely beyond control, the patient should at once seek for remedies or consult a competent physician. When blood stains are produced, then medical aid must be sought at once.

Home Treatment

Sleep in a hard bed, and rise early and take a sponge bath in cold water every morning. Eat light suppers and refrain from eating late in the evening. Empty the bladder thoroughly before retiring, bathe the spine and hips with a sponge dipped in cold water.

Never sleep lying on the back.

Avoid all highly seasoned food and read good books, and keep the mind well employed. Take regular and vigorous outdoor exercise every day.

Avoid all coffee, tea, wine, beer, and all alcoholic liquors.

Don't use tobacco.

Keep the bowels free.

Use your private organs only for what your Creator intended they should be used.

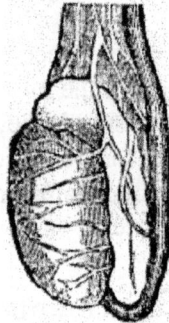

Healthy Testicle.

A Healthy Testicle

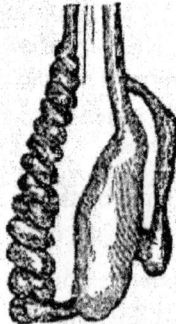

A Testicle wasted by Masturbation.

A Testicle wasted by Masturbation

Sex

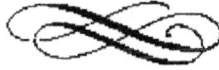

Consummation of Marriage

The first time that the husband and wife cohabit together after the ceremony has been performed is called the consummation of marriage. In most States of the U.S., and in some other countries, marriage is legally declared void and of no effect where it is not possible to consummate the marriage relation. A divorce may be obtained provide the injured party begins the suit.

Test of Virginity

The consummation of marriage with a virgin is not necessarily attended with a flow of blood, and the absence of this sign is not the slightest presumption against her former chastity. The true test of virginity is modesty void of any disagreeable familiarity. A sincere Christian faith is one of the best recommendations.

Let Every Man Remember that the legal right of marriage does not carry with it the moral right to injure for life the loving companion he has chosen

Sensuality

Lust crucifies love. The young sensual husband is generally at fault. Passion sways and the duty to bride and wife

77

is not thought of, and so a modest young wife is often actually forced and assaulted by the unsympathetic haste of her husband. An amorous man in that way soon destroys his own love, and thus is laid the foundation for many difficulties that soon develop trouble and disturb the happiness of both.

Abuse After Marriage

Usually marriage is consummated within a day or two after the ceremony, but this is gross injustice to the bride. In most cases she is nervous, timid, and exhausted by the duties of preparation for the wedding, and in no way in a condition, either in body or mind, for the vital change which the married relation brings upon her.

The First Conjugal Approaches are usually painful to the new wife, and no enjoyment to her follows. Great caution and kindness should be exercised. True love and a high regard for each other will temper passion into moderation.

A Common Error

The young husband may have read in some treatise on physiology that the hymen in a virgin is the great obstacle to be overcome. He is apt to conclude that this is all, that some force will be needed to break it down, and that therefore an amount of urgency even to the degree of inflicting considerable pain is justifiable. This is usually wrong. It rarely constitutes any obstruction, and, even when its rupturing may be necessary, it alone seldom causes suffering.

The Conditions of the Female organs depend upon the state of the mind just as much as in the case of the husband. The male, however, being more sensual, is more quickly roused. She is far less often or early ready. In its unexcited state the vagina is lax, its walls are closed together, and their surfaces covered by but little lubrication secretion. This, then, is the time for all approaches by the husband to be of the most quietest and softest demeanor, with gentle and re-assuring words, are all that should be attempted at first. The wedding day has probably been one of fatigue, and it is foolish to go farther.

When that Moment Arrives when the bride finds she can repose perfect confidence in the kindness of her husband, that his love is not purely animal, and that no violence will be attempted, the power of her affection for him will surely assert itself; the mind will act on those organs which nature has endowed to fulfill the law of their being, the walls of the vagina will expand, and the glands at the entrance will be fully lubricated by a secretion of mucus which renders congress a matter of comparative ease.

When This Responsive Enlargement and lubrication are fully realized, it is made plain why the haste and force so common to first and subsequent coition is, as it has been justly called, nothing but "legalized rape." Young husband! Prove your manhood, not by yielding to unbridled lust and cruelty, but by the exhibition of true power in self-control and patience with the helpless being confided to your care! Prolong the delightful season of courting into and through wedded life, and rich shall be your reward.

Proper Intercourse

Young husbands should wait for an invitation to the banquet, and they will be amply paid by the very pleasure sought. Invitation or permission delights, and possession by force degrades.

Sexual Proprieties and Improprieties

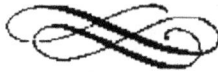

Separate Beds

Sleeping together is natural and cultivates true affection, and it is physiologically true that in very cold weather life is prolonged by husband and wife sleeping together. But in case of pregnancy, the practice of separate beds for husband and wife, will add rest to the mother and add vigor to the unborn child.

The Time for Indulgence

Intercourse should be absolutely avoided just before or after meals, or just after mental excitement or physical exercise. No wife should indulge her husband when he under the influence of alcoholic stimulants, for idiocy and other serious maladies are liable to be visited upon the offspring.

Miscarriage

If a woman is liable to abortion or miscarriage, absolute abstinence is the only remedy. No sexual indulgence during pregnancy can be safely tolerated.

Sexual Temperance

All excesses and absurdities of every kind should be carefully avoided. Many of the female disorders which often revenge themselves in the cessation of all sexual pleasure are largely due to the excessive practice of sexual indulgence.

Frequency

Some writers claim that intercourse should never occur except for the purpose of childbearing; but such restraint is not natural and consequently not conducive to health. It is now held that it is nearer a crime than a virtue to prostitute woman to the degradation of breeding animals by compelling her to bring into life more offspring than can be born healthy, or be properly cared for and educated.

A man should not gratify his own desires at the expense of his wife's health, comfort or inclination. Many men no doubt harass their wives and force many burdens upon their slender constitutions. But it is a great sin and true husband will demand unreasonable recognition. The wife when physically able, however, should bear with her husband. Man is naturally sensitive on this subject, and it takes but little to alienate his affections and bring discord into the family.

General Rule to follow

Sexual indulgence should only occur about once in a week or ten days, and this of course applies only to those who enjoy a fair degree of health. But it is a hygienic and physiological fact that those who indulge only once a month receive a far greater degree of the intensity of enjoyment than those who indulge their passions more frequently.

Chapter Eight

Female Hygiene and Disorders

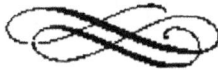

Menstruation

Menstruation - "the periods" - the appearance of the catamenia or the menses - is then one of the most important epochs in a girl's life. It is the boundary-line, the landmark between childhood and womanhood; it is the threshold, so to speak, of a woman's life. Her body now develops and expands, and her mental capacity enlarges and improves.

Menstruation in this country usually commences at the ages of from thirteen to sixteen, sometimes earlier; occasionally as early as eleven or twelve; at other times later, and not until a girl be seventeen or eighteen years of age. Menstruation in large towns is supposed to commence at an earlier period than in the country, and earlier in luxurious than in simple life.

The menstrual fluid is not exactly blood, although, both in appearance and properties, it much resembles it; yet it never in the healthy state clots as blood does. It is a secretion of the womb, and, when healthy, ought to be of a bright red color, in appearance very much like the blood from a recently cut finger. The menstrual fluid ought not, as before observed, clot. If it does, a lady, during "her periods", suffers intense pain; moreover, she seldom conceives until the clotting has ceased.

Some ladies, though comparatively few, menstruate during nursing; when they do, it may be considered not as the rule, but as the exception. It is said in such instances, that they are more likely to conceive; and no doubt they are, as menstruation is an indication of a proneness to conception. Many persons have an idea that when a woman, during lactation, menstruates, her milk is both sweeter and purer. Such is an error. Menstruation during nursing is more likely to weaken the mother, and consequently to deteriorate her milk, and thus make it less sweet and less pure.

During "the monthly periods" violent exercise is injurious; iced drinks and acid beverages are improper; and bathing in the sea, and bathing the feet in cold water, and cold baths are dangerous; indeed, at such times as these, no risks should be run, and no experiments should, for one moment, be permitted, otherwise serious consequences will, in all probability, ensue.

Vaginal Cleanliness

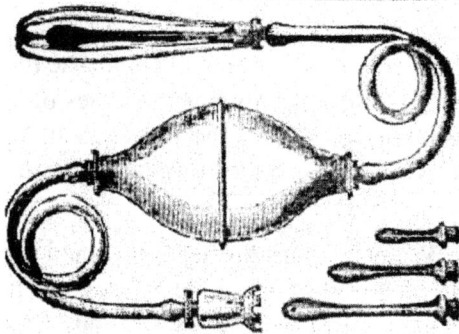

*New Revelation for Women.

A hint to the wise is sufficient. The vagina should be cleansed with the same faithfulness as any other portion of the body.

Those not accustomed to use vaginal injections would do well to use water milkwarm at the commencement; after this the temperature may be varied according to circumstances. In case of local inflammation use hot water. The indiscriminate use of cold water injections will be found rather injurious than beneficial, and a woman in feeble health will always find warm water invigorating and preferable.

The cleanser will greatly stimulate the health and spirits of any woman who uses it. Pure water injections have a stimulating effect, and it seems to invigorate the entire body.

Salt and water injections will cure cases of leucorrhoea.

Add a teaspoonful of salt to a pint and a half of water at the proper temperature. Injections may be repeated daily if deemed necessary.

Soap and water is a very simple domestic remedy, and will many times afford relief in many diseases of the womb. It seems it thoroughly cleanses the parts. A little borax or vinegar may be used the same as salt water injections.

Sterile Women desiring offspring should seek sexual union soon after the appearance of the menses, and not use the vaginal cleanser till several days later. Those not desiring offspring should avoid copulation until the ovum has passed the generative tract.

Injections during the monthly flow

Of course, it is not proper to arrest the flow, and the injections will stimulate a healthy action of the organs. The injections may be used daily throughout the monthly flow with much comfort and benefit. If the flow is scanty and painful the injections may be as warm as they can be comfortably borne. If the flowing is immoderate then cool water may be used. A woman will soon learn her own condition and can act accordingly.

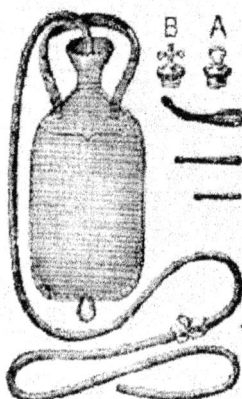

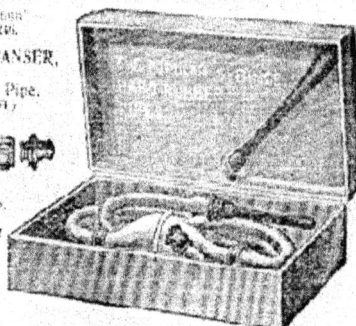

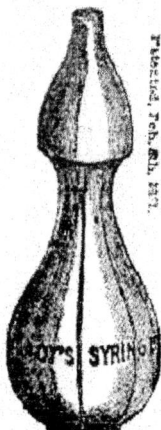

Safe Counsel

Disorders of the Menses

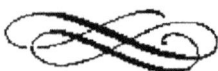

Suppression of, or Scanty Menses:

Attention to the diet, and exercise in the open air to promote the general health. Some bitter tonic taken with fifteen grains of dialyzed iron, well diluted, after meals if patient is pale and debilitated. A hot foot bath is often all that is necessary.

Profuse Menstruation:

Avoid highly seasoned food and the use of spirituous liquors; also excessive fatigue, either physical or mental. To check the flow patient should be kept quiet and allowed to sip cinnamon tea during the period.

Painful Menstruation:

Often brought on by colds. Treat by warm hip baths, hot drinks, (avoiding spirituous liquors) and heat applied to the back and extremities. A teaspoonful of the fluid extract of viburnum will sometimes act like a charm.

Miscellaneous Complaints

How to cure Swelled and Sore Breasts

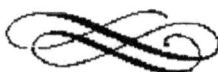

Take and boil a quantity of chamomile and apply the hot fomentations; this dissolves the knot and reduces the swelling and soreness.

Leucorrhea or Whites

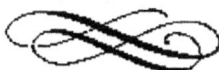

This disorder, if not arising from some abnormal condition of the pelvic organs, can easily be cured by patient taking the proper amount of exercise and good nutritious food, avoiding tea and coffee. An injection every evening of one teaspoonful of Pond's Extract in a cup of hot water, after first cleansing the vagina well with a quart of warm water, is a simple but effective remedy.

Inflammation of the Womb

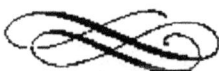

When in the acute form this disease is ushered in by a chill followed by fever, and pain in the region of the womb. Patient should be placed in bed and a brisk purgative given. Hot poultices applied to the abdomen, and the feet and hands kept warm. If the symptoms do not subside, a physician should be consulted.

Hysteria

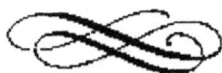

A functional disorder of the nervous system of which it is impossible to speak definitely; characterized by disturbance of the reason, will, imagination and emotions, with sometimes convulsive attacks that resemble epilepsy.

Fits of laughter, and tears without apparent cause. Emotions easily excited; mind often melancholy and depressed. Tenderness along the spine, disturbances of digestion, with hysterical convulsions, and other nervous phenomena.

Some healthy and pleasant employment should be urged upon women afflicted with this disease. Men are also subject to it, though not so frequently. Avoid excessive fatigue and mental worry; also stimulants and opiates. Plenty of good food and fresh air will do more good than drugs.

Falling of the Womb

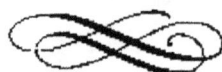

The displacement of the womb usually is the result of too much childbearing, miscarriages, abortions, or the taking of strong medicines to bring about menstruation. it may also be the result in getting up too quickly from the childbed. There are, however, other causes, such as a general breaking down of the health.

If the womb has fallen forward it presses against the bladder, causing the patient to urinate frequently. If the womb has fallen back, it presses against the rectum, and constipation is the result with often severe pain at stool. If the womb descends into the vagina there is a feeling of heaviness. All forms of displacement produce pain in the back, with an irregular and scanty menstrual flow and a dull and exhausted feeling.

Improve the general health. Take some preparation of cod-liver oil, hot injections (of a teaspoonful of powdered alum with a pint of water), a daily sitz-bath, and a regular morning bath three times a week will be found very beneficial. There, however, can be no remedy unless the womb is first replaced to the proper position. This must be done by a competent physician who should frequently be consulted.

Chapter Nine:

Dictionary of Medical Terms

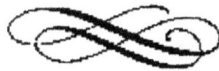

- **Abdomen** - The largest cavity of the body, containing the liver, stomach, intestines, etc.

- **Abnormal** - Unhealthy, unnatural.

- **Abortion** - A premature birth, or miscarriage.

- **Abscess** - A cavity containing pus.

- **Acetic** - Sour, acid.

- **Acidity** - Sourness.

- **Acrid** - Irritating, biting.

- **Acute** - Of short duration.

- **Adipose** - Fatty.

- **Albumen** - An animal substance resembling white of egg.

- **Alimentary Canal** - The entire passage through which food passes; the whole intestines from mouth to anus.

- **Alterative** - Medicines which gradually restore healthy action

- **Amenorrhoea** - Suppression of the menses.

- **Amorphous** - Irregular.

- **Anemia** - Bloodlessness.

- **Anesthetics** - Medicines depriving of sensation and suffering.

- **Anatomy** - Physical structure.

- **Anodyne** - A remedy used for the relief of pain.

- **Ante-natal** - Before birth.

- **Anteversion** - Bending forward.

- **Antidote** - A medicine counteracting poison.

- **Anti-emetic** - That which will stop vomiting.

- **Antiseptic** - That which will prevent putrefaction.

- **Anus** - Circular opening or outlet of the bowels.

- **Aorta** - The great artery of the heart.

- **Aphtha** - Thrush; infant sore mouth.

- **Aqua** - Water.

- **Arcola** - Circle around the nipple.

- **Astringent** - Binding; contracting.

- **Auricle** - A cavity of the heart.

- **Axilla** - The armpit.

- **Azote** - Nitrogen.

- **Bacteria** - Infusoria; microscopical insects.

- **Bicuspid** - A two-pointed tooth.

- **Bile** - Secretion from the liver.

- **Bilious** - An undue amount of bile.

- **Bronchitis** - Inflammation of the bronchial tubes which lead into the lungs.

- **Calculus** - A stone found in the bladder, gall-ducts and kidneys.

- **Callous** - A hard bony substance or growth.

- **Capillaries** - Hair-like vessels that convey the blood from the arteries to the veins.

- **Carbonic Acid** - The gas which is expired from the lungs.

- **Cardiac** - Relating to the heart.

- **Catarrh** - Flow of mucus.

- **Cathartic** - An active purgative.

- **Caustic** - A corroding or destroying substance.

- **Cellular** - Composed of cells.

- **Cervix** - Neck.

- **Cervix Uteri** - Neck of the womb.

- **Chronic** - Of long standing.

- **Clavicle** - The collar bone.

- **Coccyx** - Terminal bone of the spine.

- **Condiment** - That which gives relish to food.

- **Congestion** - Overfullness of blood vessels.

- **Contusion** - A bruise.

- **Cuticle** - The outer skin.

- **Dentition** - Act of cutting teeth.

- **Diagnosis** - Scientific determination of diseases.

- **Diarrhea** - Looseness of the bowels.

- **Disinfectant** - That which cleanses or purifies.

- **Diaphragm** - Breathing muscle between chest and abdomen.

- **Duodenum** - The first part of the small intestines.

- **Dyspepsia** - Difficult digestion.

- **Dysuria** - Difficult or painful urination.

- **Emetic** - Medicines which produce vomiting.

- **Enamel** - Covering of the teeth.

- **Enema** - An injection by the rectum.

- **Enteritis** - Inflammation of the intestines.

- **Epidemic** - Generally prevailing.

- **Epidermis** - Outer skin.

- **Epigastruim** - Region of the pit of the stomach.

- **Epilepsy** - Convulsions.

- **Eustachian Tube** - A tube leading from the side of the throat to the internal ear.

- **Evacuation** - Discharging by stool.

- **Excretion** - That which is thrown off.

- **Expectorant** - Tending to produce free discharge from the lungs or throat.

- **Fallopian Tubes** - Tubes from ovaries to uterus.

- **Fauces** - The upper part of the throat.

- **Feces** - Discharge from the bowels.

- **Fetus** - The child in the womb after the fifth month.

- **Fibula** - The smallest bone of the leg below the knee.

- **Fistula** - An ulcer.

- **Flatulence** - Gas in the stomach or bowels.

- **Flooding** - Uterine hemorrhage.

- **Fluor Albus** - White flow; leucorrhea; whites.

- **Flux** - Diarrhea, or other excessive discharge.

- **Fomentation** - Warm or hot application to the body.

- **Friable** - Easily crumbled or broken.

- **Friction** - Rubbing with the dry hand or dry coarse cloth.

- **Fumigate** - To smoke a room, or any article needing to be cleansed.

- **Function** - The office or duty of any organ.

- **Fundament -** The anus.

- **Fungus** - Spongy flesh in wounds; proud flesh.

- **Fusion** - To melt by heat.

- **Gall** - Bile.

- **Gall-Stones** - Hard biliary concretions found in the gall bladder.

- **Gangrene** - The first stage of mortification.

- **Gargle** - A liquid preparation for washing the throat.

- **Gastric** - Of the stomach.

- **Gastritis** - Inflammation of the stomach.

- **Gelatinous** - Like jelly.

- **Genitals** - The sexual organs.

- **Genu** - The knee.

- **Genus** - Family of plants; a group.

- **Germ** - the vital principal, or life spark.

- **Gestation** - Period of growth of child in the womb.

- **Gleet** - Chronic gonorrhea.

- **Glottis** - The opening of the windpipe.

- **Gonorrhea** - An infectious discharge from the genital organs.

- **Gout** - Painful inflammation of the joints of the toes.

- **Gravel** - Crystalline sand-like particles in the urine.

- **Guttural** - Relating to the throat.

- **Hectic** - A fever which occurs generally at night.

- **Hemorrhage** - A discharge of blood.

100

- **Hemorrhoids** - Piles; tumors in the anus.

- **Hepatic** - Pertaining to the liver.

- **Hereditary** - Transmitted from parents.

- **Hernia** - Rupture which permits a part of the bowels to protrude.

- **Hygiene** - Preserving health by diet and other precautions.

- **Hymen** - A membrane situated near the opening of the vagina in virgins.

- **Hyperemia** - Excess of blood in any part.

- **Hysteritis** - Inflammation of the uterus.

- **Impregnation** - The act of producing.

- **Incision** - The cutting with instruments.

- **Incontinence** - Not being able to hold the natural secretions.

- **Influenza** - A disease affecting the nostrils and throat.

- **Infusion** - The liquor in which plants have been steeped, and their medicinal virtues extracted.

- **Inhalation** - Drawing in the breath.

- **Injection** - Any preparation introduced into the rectum or other cavity by syringe.

- **Inspiration** - The act of drawing air into the lungs.

- **Insomnia** - Sleeplessness.

- **Involuntary** - Against the will.

- **Introversion** - Against the will.

- **Jaundice** - A disease caused by the inactivity of the liver or ducts leading from it.

- **Jugular** - Belonging to the throat.

- **Kidneys** - Two organs which secrete the urine.

- **Labia** - The lips of the vagina.

- **Laryngitis** - Inflammation of the throat.

- **Larynx** - The upper part of the throat.

- **Lassitude** - Weakness; a feeling of stupor.

- **Laxative** - Remedy increasing action of the bowels.

- **Leucorrhoea** - whites; fluor albis.

- **Livid** - A dark colored spot on the surface.

- **Loin** - Lower part of the back.

- **Lotion** - A preparation to wash a sore.

- **Lumbago** - Rheumatism of the loins.

- **Malaria** - Foul marsh air.

- **Malignant** - A disease of a very serious character.

- **Malformation** - Irregular, unnatural formation.

- **Mastication** - The act of chewing.

- **Masturbation** - Excitement, by the hand, of the genital organs.

- **Matrix** - the womb.

- **Meconium** - The first passage of babes after birth.

- **Membrane** - A thin lining or covering.

- **Menopause** - Change of life.

- **Menstruation** - Monthly discharge of blood from the uterus.

- **Midwifery** - Art of assisting at childbirth.

- **Mucus** - A fluid secreted or poured out by the mucous membrane, serving to protect it.

- **Narcotic** - A medicine relieving pain and producing sleep.

- **Nephritis** - Inflammation of the kidneys.

- **Neuralgia** - Pain in nerves.

- **Nocturnal** - Occurring in the night.

- **Normal** - In a natural condition.

- **Nutritious** - A substance which feeds the body.

- **Obesity** - Excess of fat or flesh.

- **Obstetrics** - The science of midwifery.

- **Oculous** - The eye.

- **Oesophagus** - The tube leading from the throat to the stomach.

- **Optic Nerve** - The nerve which enters the back part of the eye.

- **Organic** - Having organs.

- **Os** - Mouth; used as mouth of womb.

- **Ostalgia** - Inflammation of the ear.

- **Ovum** - An egg.

- **Oxalic Acid** - An acid found in sorrel, very poisonous.

- **Palate** - The roof of the mouth.

- **Palliative** - To afford relief only.

- **Palpitation** - Unnatural beating of the heart.

- **Paralysis** - Loss of motion.

- **Parturition** - Childbirth.

- **Pathological** - Morbid, diseased.

- **Pelvis** - The bony cavity at lower part of trunk.

- **Pericardium** - Sac containing the heart.

- **Perineum** - The floor of the pelvis, or space between and including the anus and vulva.

- **Peritonitis** - Inflammation of lining membrane of bowels.

- **Placenta** - After birth.

- **Pleura** - Membrane covering the lungs.

- **Pleurisy** - Inflammation of the pleura.

- **Pregnancy** - Being with child.

- **Prognosis** - Prediction of termination of a disease.

- **Prolapsus** - Falling; protrusion.

- **Prolapsus Uteri** - Falling of the womb.

- **Prostration** - without strength.

- **Pruritis** - A skin trouble causing intense itching.

- **Puberty** - Full growth.

- **Pubes** - External part of the organs of generation covered with hair.

- **Puerperal** - Belonging to childbirth.

- **Pulmonary** - Pertaining to the lungs.

- **Pulmonitis** - Inflammation of the lungs.

- **Pus** - Unhealthy matter.

- **Putrid** - Rotten, decomposed.

- **Pylorus** - Lower opening of the stomach.

- **Rectum** - The lower portion of the intestines.

- **Regimen** - Regulated habits and food.

- **Renal** - Pertaining to the kidneys.

- **Retching** - An effort to vomit.

- **Retina** - Inner coat of the eye.

- **Retroversion** - Falling backward.

- **Rigor** - Chilliness, convulsive shuddering.

- **Sacrum** - Bone of the pelvis.

- **Saliva** - Fluid of the mouth.

- **Salivation** - Unnatural flow of saliva.

- **Sanative** - Health producing.

- **Sciatic** - Pertaining to the hip.

- **Scrofula** - A constitutional tendency to disease of the glands.

- **Scrotum** - The sac which encloses the testicles.

- **Sedative** - Quieting, soothing.

- **Semen** - Secretion of the testes.

- **Sitz-bath** - Bath in a sitting position.

- **Sterility** - Barrenness.

- **Stimulant** - A medicine calculated to excite an increased and healthy action.

- **Styptic** - A substance to stop bleeding.

- **Sudorific** - Inducing sweat.

- **Tampon** - A plug to arrest hemorrhage.

- **Tonic** - A medicine which increases the strength of the system.

- **Testicle** - Gland that secretes the semen.

- **Therapeutic** - Treatment of disease.

- **Tissue** - The peculiar structure of a part.

- **Tonsils** - Glands on each side of the throat.

- **Trachea** - Windpipe.

- **Triturate** - To rub into a powder.

- **Tumor** - A morbid enlargement of a part.

- **Ulceration** - The forming of an ulcer.

- **Umbilicus** - The navel.

- **Ureter** - Duct leading from the bladder.

- **Uterus** - The womb.

- **Vagina** - The passage from the womb to the vulva.

- **Varicose Veins** - Veins dilated with accumulation of dark colored blood.

- **Vascular** - Relating to the blood vessels.

- **Vena Cava** - The large vein communicating with the heart.

- **Venous** - Pertaining to the veins.

- **Ventricle** - One of the lower chambers of the heart.

- **Viable** - Capable of life.

- **Vulva** - Outer lips of the vagina.

- **Womb** - That organ of the woman which conceives and nourishes the offspring.

- **Zymotic** - Caused by fermentation.

Chapter Ten

Old Disease Names & Their Modern Definitions

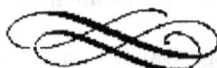

- **Acute Mania** - severe insanity

- **Addison's Disease** - a destructive disease marked by weakness, loss of weight, low blood pressure, gastrointestinal disturbances, and brownish pigmentation of the skin and mucous membranes.

- **Aphonia** - laryngitis

- **Apoplexy** - stroke

- **Ague** - used to define the recurring fever & chills of malarial infection

- **Biliousness** - jaundice or other symptoms associated with liver disease

- **Black Jaundice (Wiel's Disease)** - Black jaundice is a common term for Wiel's Disease. It is quite common in northeast England near mines, farms and sewage and floats about in water. It is caused by a micro-organism and thus is a bacterial infection (of the liver) and not a virus, as in hepatitis. It is carried by rats and secreted in their urine. It is usually not fatal, in present time, to humans. It is, however, rapidly fatal to dogs and cats, who can eventually gain a resistance, but either way can pass it on.

· **Bright's Disease** - Bright's Disease is a catch-all for kidney diseases/disorders

· **Camp Fever** - typhus

· **Canine Madness** - hydrophobia

· **Carditis** - inflammation of the heart wall

· **Catarrh** - inflammation of mucous membrane

· **Chlorosis** - iron deficency anemia

· **Chorea (St. Vitus' Dance)** - nervous disorder

· **Commotion** - Concussion

· **Consumption** - tuberculosis

· **Corruption** - infection

· **Coryza** - a cold

· **Costiveness** - constipation

· **Cramp Colic** - appendicitis

· **Croup** - spasmodic laryngitis esp. of infants, marked by episodes of difficult breathing and hoarse metallic cough

· **Death from "teething"** - tooth infections with inflammation and cellulitis were clearly important causes of illness and death before there was adequate dentistry.

· **Domestic Illness** - polite way of saying mental breakdown, depression, Alzheimers, Parkinsons, or the after effects of a stroke or any illness that kept a person housebound and probably in need of nursing support.

· **Dropsy** - edema (swelling), often caused by kidney or heart disease. Dropsy would be called congestive heart failure today. It is an accumulation of fluid around the heart, for a variety of complex reasons, and one treatment is administration of digitalis (foxglove leaves).

- **Dyspepsia** - acid indigestion

- **Extravastaed blood** - rupture of a blood vessel

- **Falling Sickness** - epilepsy

- **Flux of Humour** - circulation

- **French Pox** - veneral disease a

- **Gout** - any inflammation, not just in a joint or extremity, caused by the formation of crystals of oxalic acid when it accumulates in the body. It most often occurs in joints where circulation is poor, and can even cause gallstones or kidney stones. Gout is a disease caused by a buildup of urate or uric acid in the body, which crystallizes out in areas without much rapid blood flow and can cause damage when, for example a toe is stubbed.

- **Green Sickness** - anemia

- **Hip Gout** - osteomylitis

- **Jail Fever** - typhus

- **King's Evil (Scrofula)** - tubercular infection of the throat lymph glands

- **La Grippe** - flu

- **Lues** - syphilis.

- **Lues Venera** - veneral disease

- **Lumbago** - back pain

- **Lung Fever** - pneumonia

· **Lung Sickness** - tuberculosis

· **Mania** - insanity

· **Marasmus** - progressive emaciation

· **Membranous Croup** - hoarse cough

· **Milk Leg** - a painful swelling of the leg beginning at the ankle and ascending, or at the groin and extending down the thigh. It's usual cause is infection after labor.

· **Mortification** - infection

· **Neurasthenia** - neurotic condition

· **Nostalgia** - homesickness

· **Pott's Disease** - tuberculosis of the spine with destruction of the bone resulting in curvature of the spine

· **Protein Disease** - a once relatively common childhood kidney disease that causes the kidney to leak protien. This is a secondary allergic reaction to certain kinds of strep infections.

· **Putrid Fever** - diptheria

· **Quinsy** - tonsilitis

· **Remitting Fever** - malaria

· **Sanguineous Crust** - scab

· **Screws** - rheumatism

· **Scrofula** - see King's Evil

· **Septicemia** - blood poisoning

· **Ship's Fever** - typhus

· **Strangery** - rupture

· **Summer Complaint** - dysentry or baby diarrhea caused by spoiled milk

· **Venesection (Bleeding Venesection)** - bleeding

www.ingramcontent.com/pod-product-compliance
Lightning Source LLC
Chambersburg PA
CBHW052117090426
42741CB00009B/1849